THE MYSTER...
A CORONAVIRUS EXPLORATION FOR KIDS

WRITTEN BY CHANIE CHEIN

WATERCOLOR ART BY SHAINA ROTHMAN

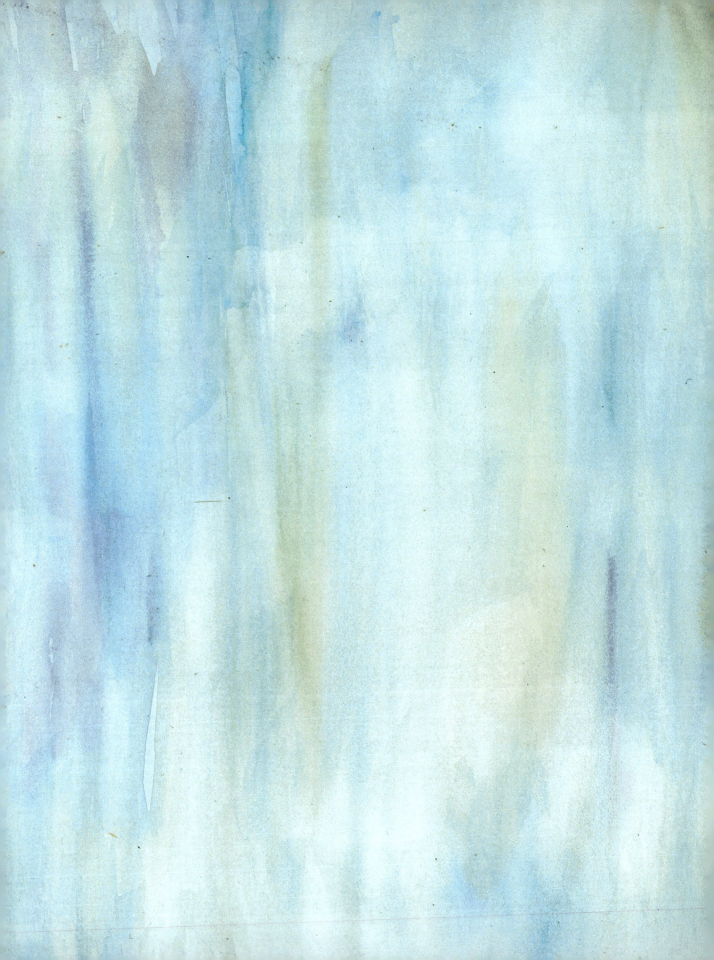

This Book Belongs To:

_____

B"H

Copyright © 2020 by Chanie (Rothman) Chein
Illustrated by Shaina Rothman

Published by Honey Pot Press
www.honeypotpress.com
info@honeypotpress.com

All rights reserved.
No part of this book may be reproduced or used in any manner whatsoever without the express written permission from the copyright holder except for the use of a brief quotation in a book review.

ISBN: **978-0-578-77530-2**

Note from the author:

Like many other schools, when the Covid 19 Coronavirus hit, our early childhood center had to shut down in-person classes and open up via ZOOM.

About two months into ZOOM classes, one child raised her hand and asked, "When can we go back to our real life? I really don't like this fake life at all!"

Realizing that I had to do something more to support the children emotionally, I sat down with a computer and this story was born.

As we eagerly await the time when the virus will be but a memory, my hope is that this book helps you and your family navigate these challenging times.

- Chanie

This book is dedicated to the kids at

Manhattan Jewish Montessori

who persevered through almost four months

of ZOOM learning when it was not safe

to be at school in-person.

Aria	Kenya
Ava	Maylo
Avital	Mia
Carson	Miriam
David	Ritta
Itta	Samantha
Jacob	Saul
Kennedy	Wendy
	William

THE MYSTERY VIRUS

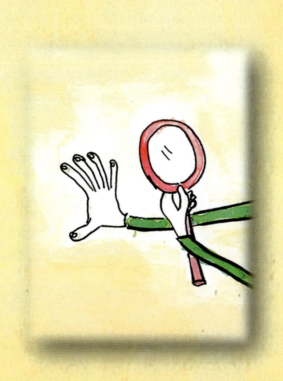

This story tells a tale of not so long ago, when suddenly everything in my world got all mixed up.

The Covid 19 Coronavirus came to town, and that meant my family and I had to stay at home.

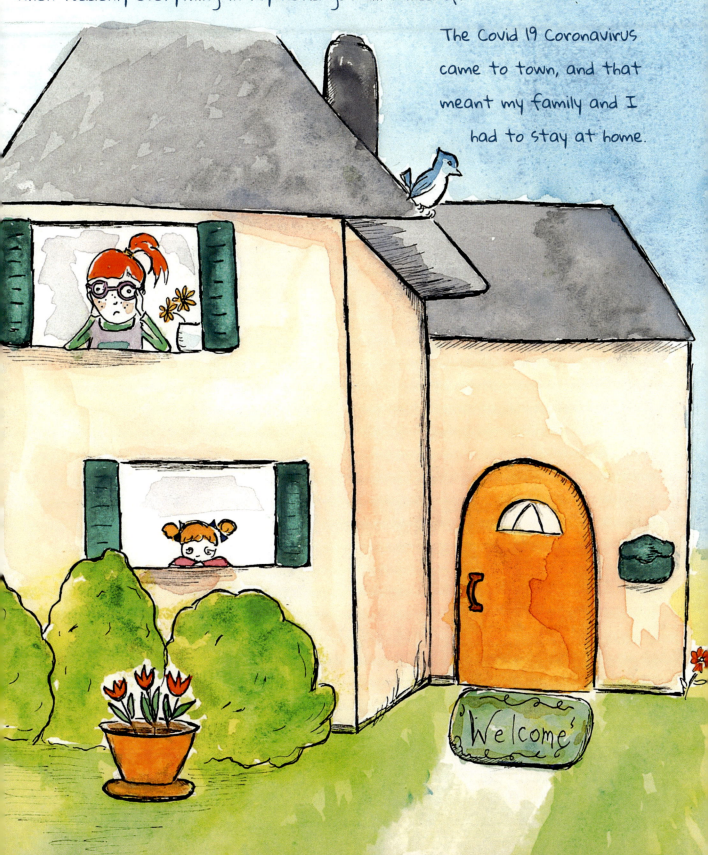

But what was the Covid 19 Coronavirus?

I decided to investigate.

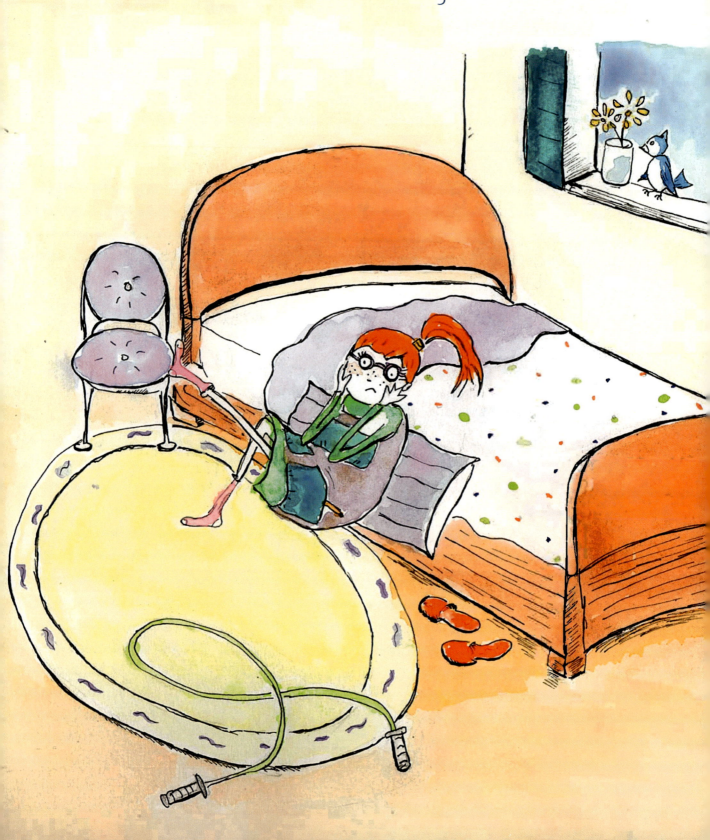

I grabbed my binoculars and ran out of my bedroom, right past my younger sister.

"Where are you going?" she called out.

"It's a Coronavirus experiment," I said. "Come with me!"

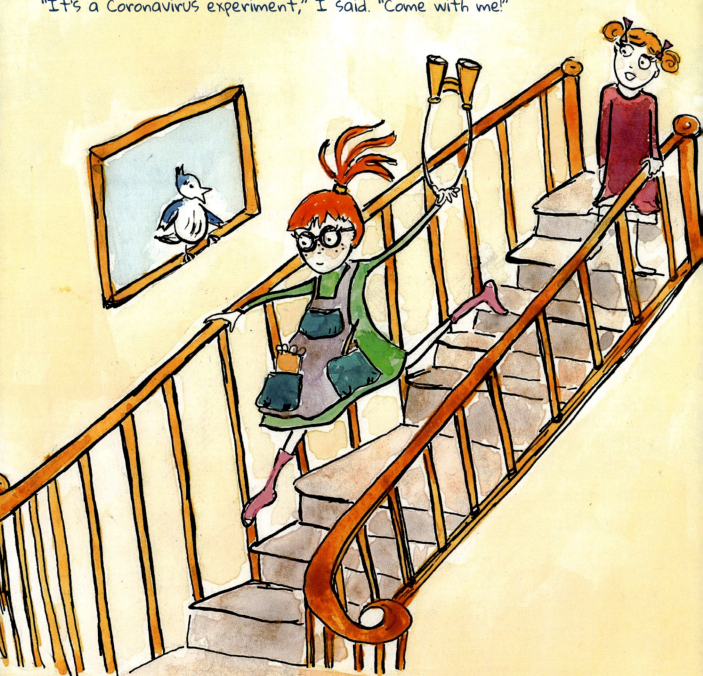

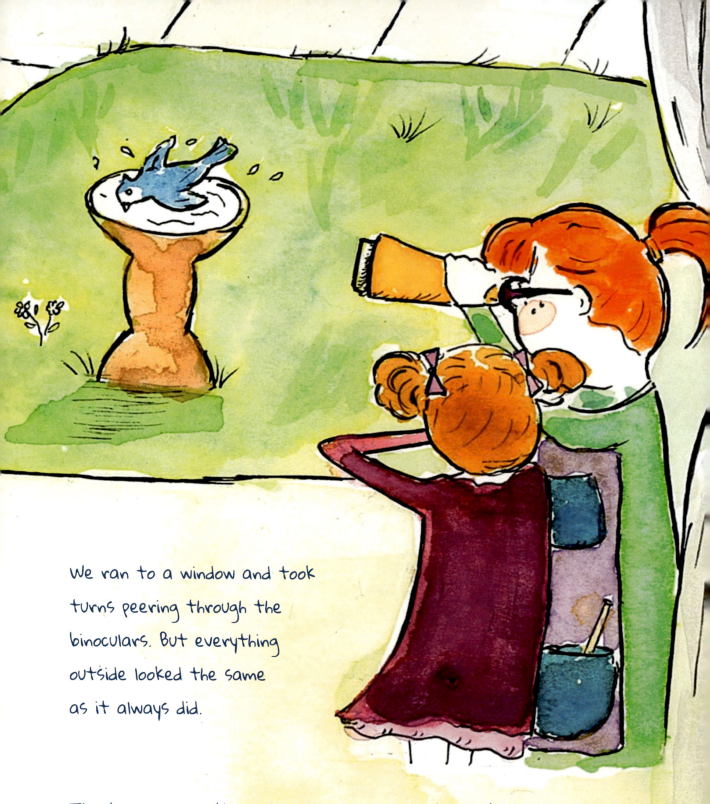

We ran to a window and took turns peering through the binoculars. But everything outside looked the same as it always did.

The trees were still green. The cars were still parked. Even the sun was shining the way it always did in spring. I didn't see the Coronavirus anywhere!

I walked back to my room and flopped onto my bed.

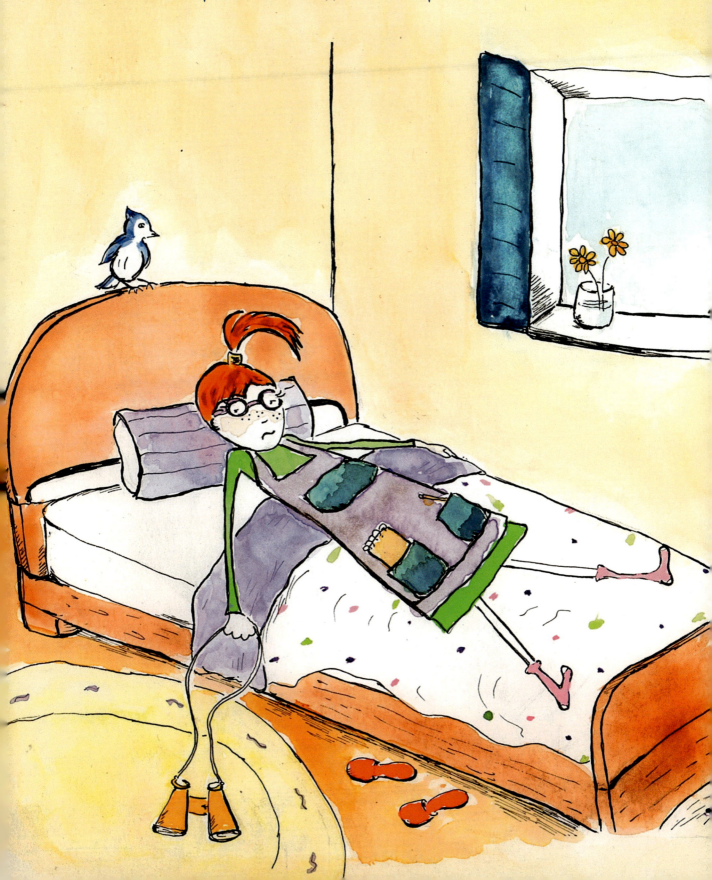

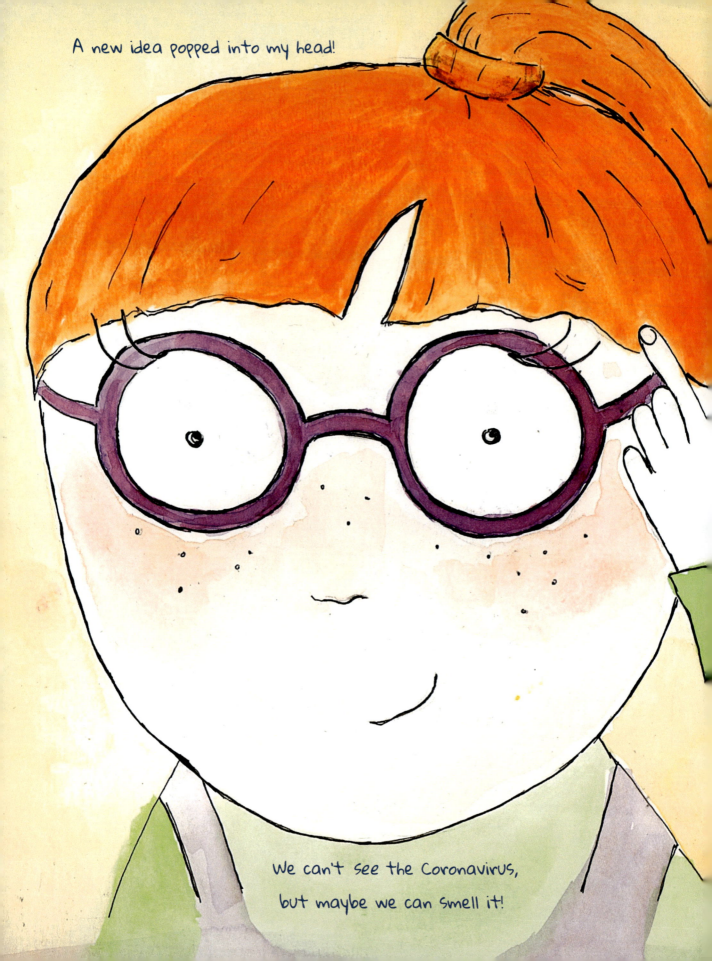

Time for a new experiment!

This time I went alone. I yanked open the back door to our house.

Then I poked my head out just a tiny bit and started to sniff around.

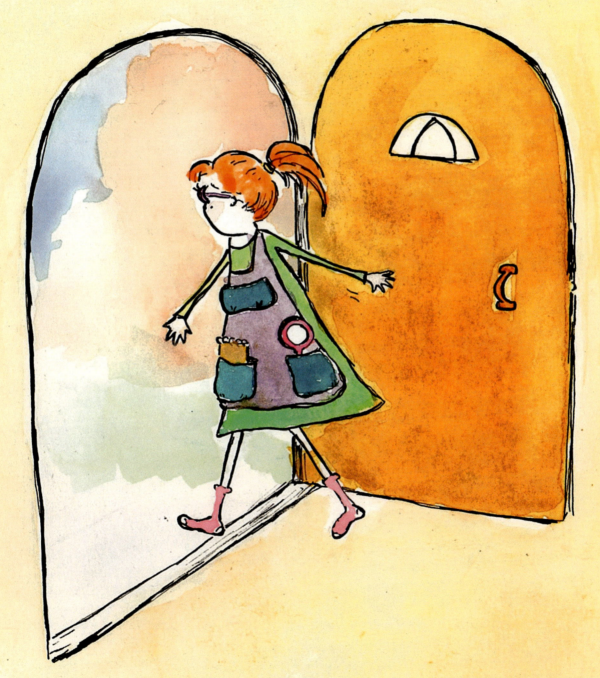

Sniff sniff, sniff sniff... nothing.

I ran to the front door. Sniff sniff, sniff sniff... still nothing!

I did not give up. I was determined to find out what this Coronavirus was all about.

I went to find a quiet place to think.

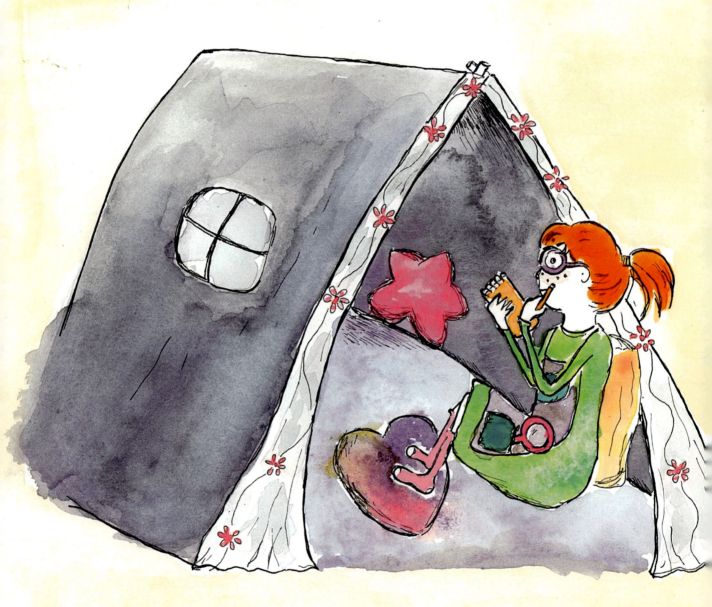

If we can't smell the Coronavirus, or see the Coronavirus, maybe we can feel it?

Time for a new experiment!

I put on my facemask, went back to the front door, and stepped outside very slowly. I looked right and then left to make sure no people were close to me. Then I stretched out my hands in front of me and began walking like a robot.

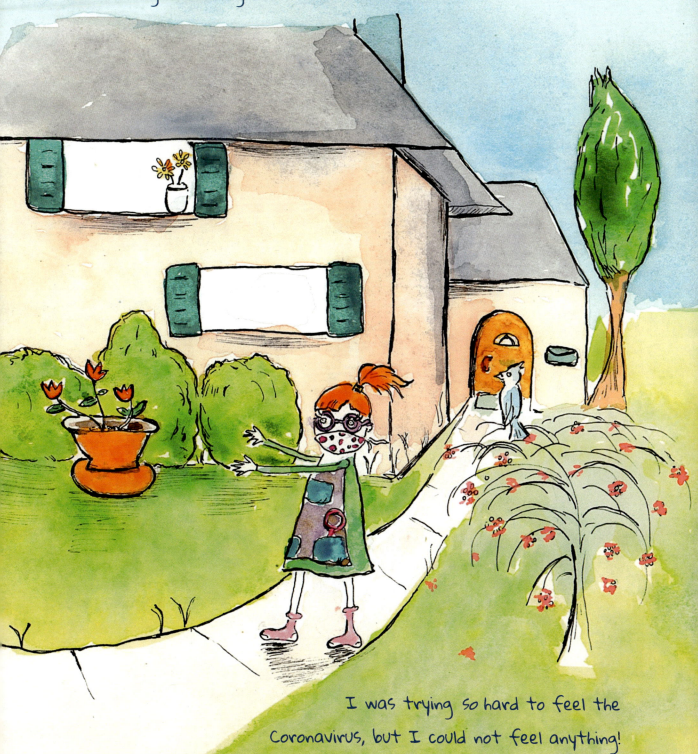

I was trying so hard to feel the Coronavirus, but I could not feel anything!

I walked back to the house and went to find a snack in the kitchen.
I was in the middle of eating when a new thought came to me!

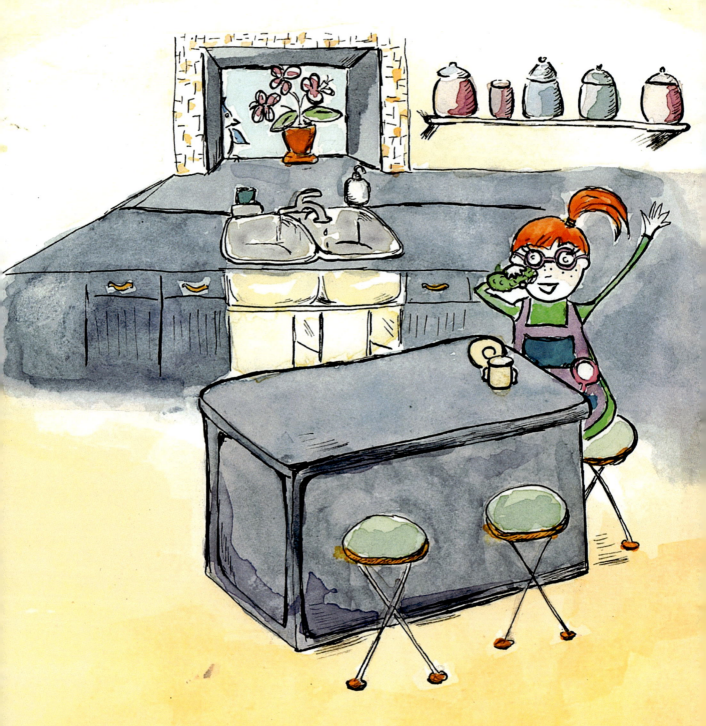

If we can't feel, or smell, or see the Coronavirus,
 maybe we can taste it! Time for a new experiment!

The kitchen window was wide open. Perfect! I opened my mouth and gulped down some fresh air. Then, I slowly licked my lips and waited.

But no taste came. There was no taste at all.

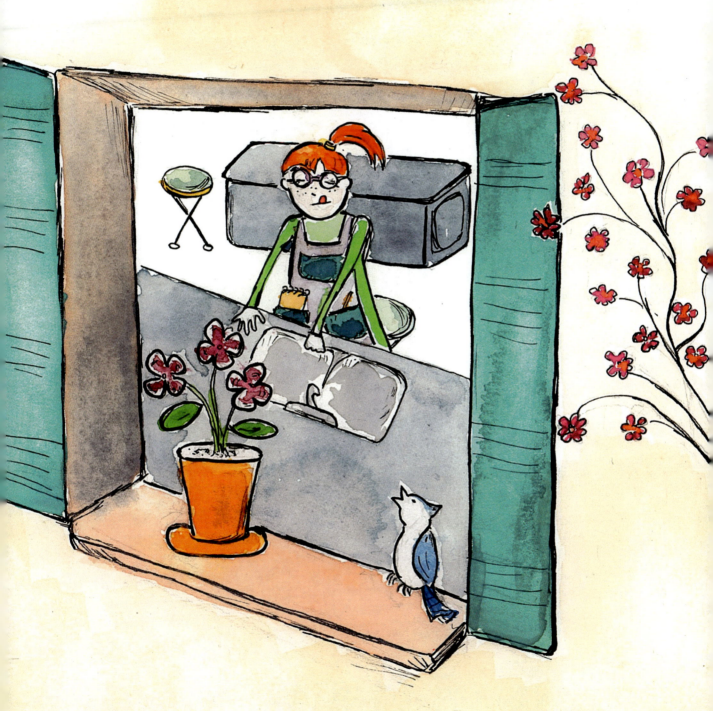

"That's strange," I said. "I already experimented with tasting, feeling, smelling, and seeing. What now?"

"What about hearing?" my sister yelled.
"Maybe you can *hear* the Coronavirus!"
How did I forget about that?

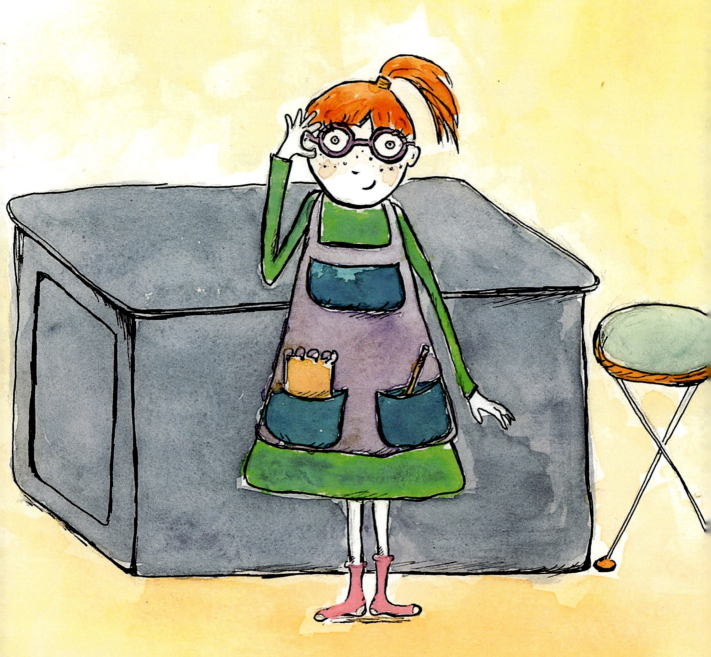

But I think I already knew the answer, and yep I was right. We definitely cannot *hear* the Coronavirus!

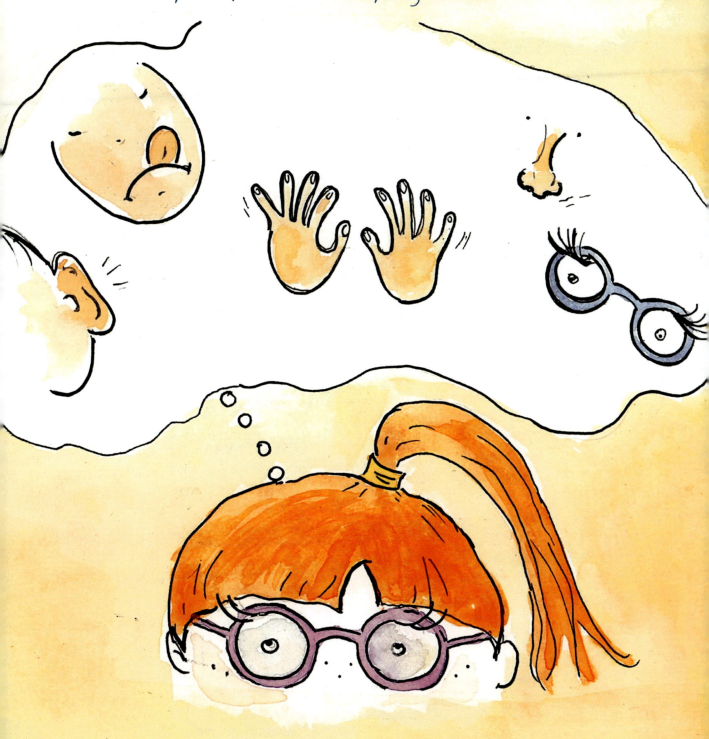

Now I was really stumped. I tried everything!

Suddenly it all became clear. If we can't *hear, taste, feel, smell,* or *see* the Coronavirus, it has to be invisible! That must be it!

I ran to find my sister, took her hands and danced around the room. I was so excited that I had finally figured it out.

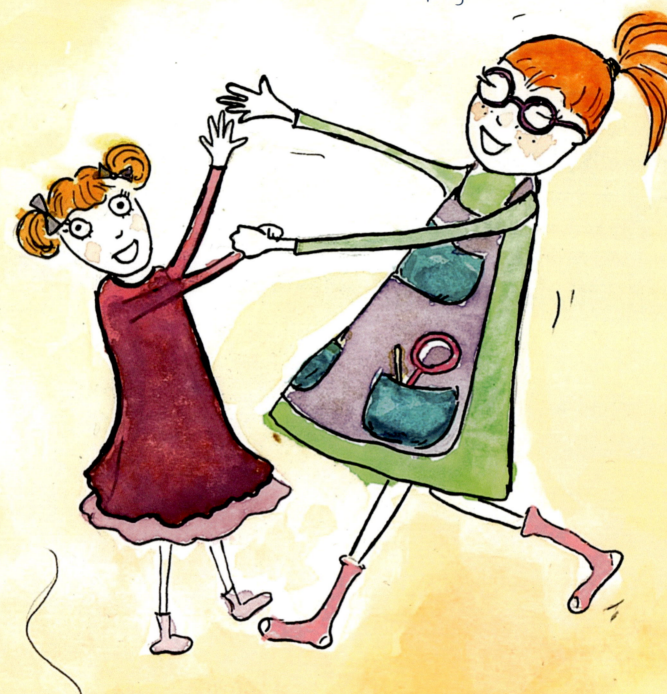

"It's invisible, it's invisible! The Coronavirus must be invisible! Mom once told me that when something is invisible, it means that it is still there, even if we can't see it!"

"You are right!" my mom called from the other room.
"The Coronavirus is made up of teeny tiny unhealthy germs that spread very quickly from one person to the next.

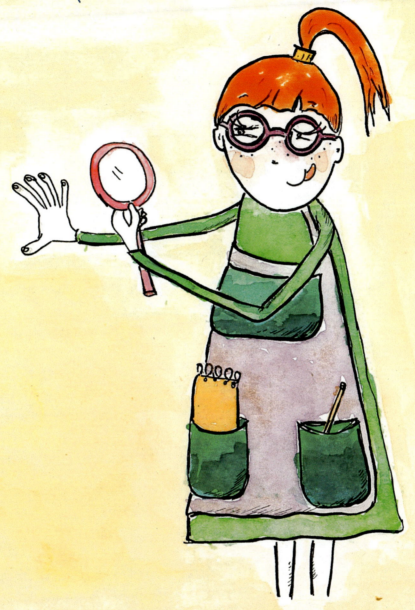

They are so teeny tiny that we can't see them, hear them, smell them, taste them, or feel them!"

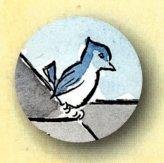

I was so relieved!

Now all the new changes in my Coronavirus life started to make sense to me!

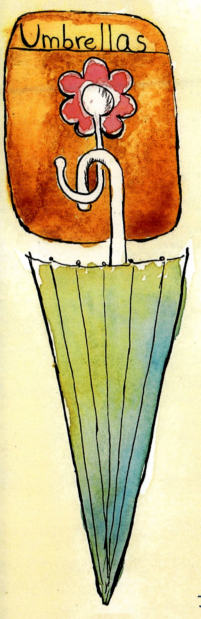
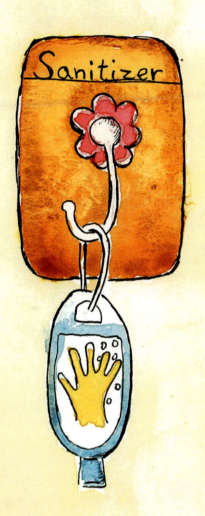
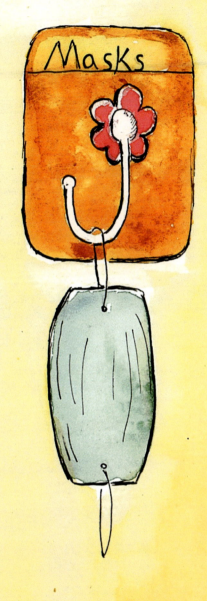

I might have to wear a mask to protect myself and other people, and I might have to stand far from my friends when I see them on the street. I know there might be other changes too, but I also know that all of the new things I am doing will help keep my body healthy.

So Covid 19 Coronavirus, I wish you would go away forever, but in the meantime I will be sure to take care of myself and continue to explore.

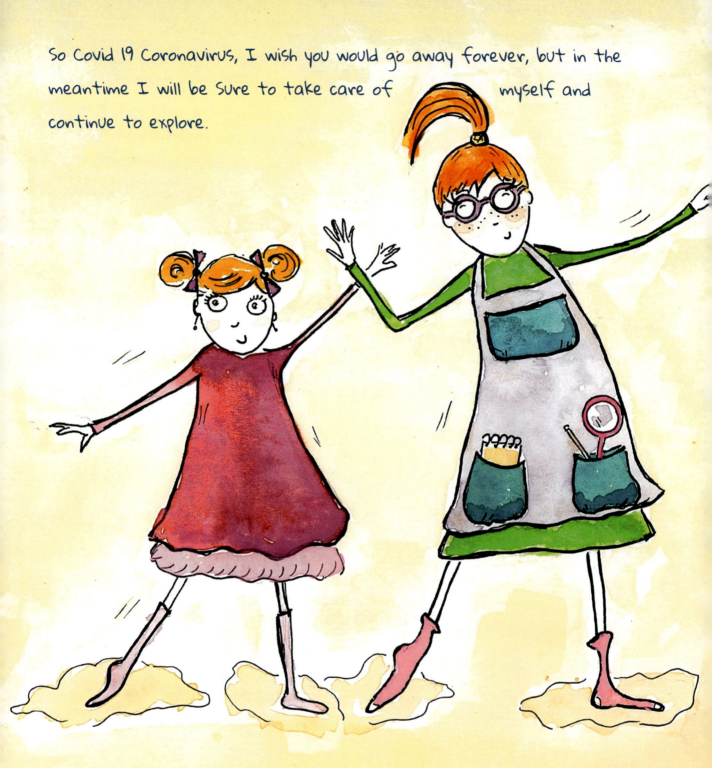

And while I am doing all of that, I will also dream for my world to go back to the way it was before everything got all mixed up.

THE END

UNTIL OUR NEXT ADVENTURE!

From the artist:

To all Rothmans everywhere and anywhere; keep on asking!

To my husband, our children, and Vicki; thank you for making it happen!

Contact the artist:
shaina.rothman@gmail.com

Made in the USA
Columbia, SC
23 October 2020